GET BACK THE MAN
WHO ROMANCED YOU

HEALTH & FITNESS

tips for a better life

TOGETHER

by

Dr. Patricia L. Skergan, D.C.

Cover design by For the Muse Designs

Edited by Clare Wood, Self-Publishing Services LLC (www.Self-Publishing-Service.com)

Formatted by Self-Publishing Services LLC

Has Your Man's "get up and go" gone?
Three life-changing strategies you can implement
for your guy to look and feel better.

CHAPTER 1

"Aliens impregnate men over forty at Deer Lodge, Montana, truck stop. Babies due any day."

When stopping to use the truck stop restroom, I thought this was going to be the headline in the local paper tomorrow. Every man I saw looked distorted in form. They all looked like they were nine months pregnant and ready to give birth. In reality, though, they were all grossly out of shape. Is this what men of today look like? Was I looking at a local phenomenon, or is this male malformation common nationwide?

Half Moon Bay is an upscale seaside town outside of San Francisco. On a recent trip I thought, "Wow, California, major metropolitan area, the guys have to be in better shape than Deer Lodge, Montana." Well, they may have been better groomed, and had fewer nose and ear hairs, but many of the guys had that distinctive belly, poor posture, and gloomy patina.

What is happening to the men in our culture? Why are all these guys so obese and looking so miserable? I'm sure they weren't born this way, so what happened? Why? When?

How? Is it progressive? And, can it be reversed?

If you are one of these, or if you are married to one and want to get yourself or him back to looking and feeling better, then read on. However, if you are perfectly content with him glued to the couch and staring at the TV, which you may well be because he's not bugging you, then this book is not for you at the moment.

While this book is for and about men, I'm also directing it to women. Women in our culture still do most of the food preparation and grocery shopping. Women make ninety percent of all doctors' appointments and purchase most of the nutritional supplements. They usually decide where and when we eat out at restaurants. Women also plan most of the social functions, including parties and dinners. They are the social directors of the family, arranging most of the weekend activities and vacations. Get the picture? We are the planners![i]

Most men eat what is in front of them and take the pills set out by their partners. In my clinical practice, I'd ask what medications and supplements the men took, only to hear the same answer: "I don't know. My wife sets them out, and I take what she gives me." I'd also ask what diet they followed. "The one my wife cooks." While I don't want to stereotype genders, the statistics[ii] speak for themselves, and women, typically, are the caretakers of the men in the family. So the responsibility, just as if they were children, is yours to make sure they eat well, get proper supplements, and exercise regularly. I wish this wasn't the case and everyone over eighteen would be held accountable for themselves. But my wish is not everyone's command.

I have a friend who is happily married and a great cook. Fortunately for her husband, she is a healthy and conscientious cook. They married later in life. So you can understand why I was surprised that, when she went away for a few days, she had "prepared" all his meals ahead of time. I asked, "Okay, he didn't marry you until he was forty-five. What did he eat all those years without you?" Her reply was that he cooked for himself, and his friends said he was a pretty good cook at that. Is it apathy or advocating for stereotypical roles that causes people to give up their freedom of choice about the food they eat?

Ladies, if you are happy with the status quo of how your husband looks, feels, acts, and functions, then don't change a thing. However, you might find yourself staring at your wedding photograph and asking, "What the hell happened to him?" I know you can make a significant change in his, yours, and your family's lives. Next year at this time, you may not recognize your life due to the positive changes that have occurred. And yes, it will take time. But you will begin to notice results in at least ten days of changing some very simple but fundamental lifestyle choices.

For decades the healthcare industry has highlighted and catered to a woman's hormonal changes. The pharmaceutical companies have numerous medications to handle all the ups and downs of peri-menopause, menopause, post-menopause, hot flashes, vaginal dryness, night sweats, irritability, dry skin, breast tenderness, sleep disruptions, emotional swings, etc. There are numerous hormonal tests that women are encouraged to perform to indicate exactly which hormone is deficient and what to use to replace it. Also on the playing field are a stockpile of nutritional formulas and vitamin supplements, just in case you don't want to go the medication route. There are herbal formulas, teas, essential oils, homeopathic remedies, and bath additives to deal with these symptoms as well.

The subject of menopause in women is discussed, diagnosed, and treated in the open and even in mixed company. Advertisements on television, in newspapers, and in magazines are now commonplace. This may not have been the case fifty years ago for women, but in today's marketplace and media, when it comes to airing any type of female problem, anything goes.

But what about the men? Do they go through hormonal changes as they age? When woman go through "the change of life," it is a definitive event. Sure, menopause is a process, yet there is an exact date when menstruation ceases. From that point, there is no more buying tampons or menstrual pads. There is no more counting the twenty-eight or so days on the menstrual cycle (the red "x" on the calendar), and there are no more pregnancies. It's done, all done.

But not so for the men. Men's hormonal changes are not marked. They are very gradual, but they do occur nevertheless. With most gradual changes they cannot be readily perceived by looking for the changes from day to day or even month to month. Hormonal changes are so gradual that most people see it as "just getting older." Look, your hormones are changing, you are not dying. And you can do something about it.

The emphasis on men's hormones has, in part, led to an emphasis on only one aspect of male menopause: erectile dysfunction. But there are many other aspects to examine. Paying attention to these other aspects will not only improve a guy's sex life, but also enhance his entire health and vitality, both mental and physical.

I know this is a taboo subject. In fact, after interviewing seasoned healthcare providers, they admit that male patients are not too chatty about the subject of male menopause. Erectile dysfunction and prostate cancer may be within limits. But a whole host of other symptoms is just taken for granted as "normal" male aging, for which nothing can be done.

CHAPTER 2

What signs and symptoms do men going through "the change of life" manifest? What tests do they go for, and where are their pills, potions, and lotions? Have you seen any television commercials featuring new medications or herbal formulas for the guy who is "suffering" from symptoms of male menopause? I'm betting you haven't. In fact, I'll bet you don't know what those signs are and haven't discussed it with anyone.

So, what are we looking at in terms of symptoms? First, let's look at some categories and then break them down to be more specific. One very important thing to keep in mind when going over these symptoms is that the outward expression or manifestation can vary in degree. So just because your guy has gotten wise enough over the years not to pick a fight with a grizzly bear, that doesn't mean he has decreased competitiveness (a symptom). Or if he is grieving the loss of a loved one, that doesn't mean he's depressed or withdrawn. What you, or even better, both of you, need to do is objectively look at the whole picture, not just a few pixels.

The categories of male menopause symptoms and signs that are addressed in this book are:

- Mental and emotional
- Musculoskeletal/physical
- Sexual
- Hormonal/metabolic

CHAPTER 3

MENTAL/EMOTIONAL

Honey, are you in there?

1. *Depression*

2. *Irritability/anger*

3. *Social isolation or antisocial behavior*

4. *Decrease of the competitive edge*

5. *Insomnia and nervousness*

6. *Mental fatigue, lack of concentration,*

7. *Hopelessness, "what's the use"*

8. *Lack of spontaneity or creativity*

9. *Loss of interest in usual activities, such as sports, or hobbies*

10. *Loss of confidence, failing memory, burnout*

11. *Sullen, lacking a sense of humor*

12. *Feeling unloving and unlovable.*

Any of these ring a bell with you?

Are you getting the picture? This guy is a party downer, a bore, and a naysayer. You know the one, complaining constantly about the government, the job, the neighbors, and the economy. You name a situation, and he's got an opinion, and it's not a good one. Don't even think of making light of a subject, or Heaven forbid, telling a joke. He won't get it, and he will probably just show more signs of irritation and irritability. To make a fast break when talking to one of these guys, all you can do is ask for a specific date, time, or fact. Likely he's forgotten the fact and will space out wracking his nervous brain to find the answer. When this happens, excuse yourself politely, as not to irritate him, and walk away. But, unless you're a public worker, friend, or family member, you probably won't see or talk to him because he has few friends, doesn't go out, and really doesn't want to be bothered talking to you anyway.

Guys, generally, are not as social as women. In fact, statistics show[iii] that most men will not make any significant or new friendships after high school or college. They may have casual social acquaintances, but mostly these are people who they find themselves "thrown" in with because they are the wife's social connections. Or they will attend work functions, religious/church gatherings, or something similar. Rarely do older men plan dinner out with the guys (like a lady's night out), get together for coffee, or workout together. Thus, any examination and sharing of how or what they are feeling and what they are going through is largely non-existent.

And if you ask, you will probably just get a grunt or at most a one-word answer.

Sometimes I'll ask my husband when he comes home, "How was the office today?"

He replies, "Fine."

"And how was your guitar lesson?"

"Fine"

"And how was your exercise workout?"

"Fine."

At this point, I remember, and say, "Okay, I'm not going to ask any more about how things were because I'm psychic and already know your answer. It is going to be 'fine'!"

We don't need to judge it, but we need to take note of the social differences and notice if this social isolation escalates, especially after retirement. The significant sign is when the social contacts who have been there in the past, such as old buddies, children, grandchildren, and other groups, are now being avoided completely, or if he passively defaults to you to make all the arrangements for going out and being with others.

In addition to the social isolation, there is a lack of enthusiasm for those activities and projects that once were top priority. "New or different" is not interesting because he's in the "what's the use of trying anyway" mode. With this mindset, sitting on the couch watching the news wins again. Of course, he may say that he can't get off the couch because he is so tired due to the fact that he was up in the middle of the night or the early morning worrying over something, which could be a dwindling bank account, a fight with the cell phone carrier, back hairs, worms in the garden, the car battery, cancer, the stock market, etc.

CHAPTER 4

PHYSICAL/ MUSCULOSKELTAL ISSUES

1. *"Beer belly"*
2. *Man boobs*
3. *Love handles*
4. *Loss of muscle tone, mass, and strength*
5. *Decrease in flexibility*
6. *Soreness, stiffness and pain*
7. *Loss of endurance (stamina)*

The physical ramifications of male menopause are only outward manifestations of what, hormonally, is happening on the inside. They are effects and ought to be treated as such. Unfortunately, most men in our culture treat them as the cause. And the cause is something to be eradicated, even if it makes other symptoms worse.

It's such a vicious circle. For example, after much prodding, he finally digs in and cleans the garage. The next day, his lower back and neck are sore, he's pulled a hamstring, and that old shoulder injury is nagging him. So he'll have to sit out the Sunday outing with you and the family and stay on the couch and watch TV all day, having baloney sandwiches and beer along with eating anti-inflammatory pills like candy.

Anti-inflammatories such as NSAIDS (non-steroidal anti-inflammatory drugs like ibuprofen, acetaminophen, and aspirin) may cause a relative lowering of testosterone Do you see the cascade of behaviors that adds to the physical manifestation of this poor quality of life? Because there is already a decrease in his usual stamina, he may not want to tackle projects or play sports because he can't do or perform at the same level he used to. Thus, another vicious cycle is initiated and completed.

The physical patterns are big bellies, i.e. the "I'm due to have this kid any day and have the boobs and belly to prove it" look. Because they've given up on most, if not all, physical activity, their upper-body physique is the "little old man" posture, with shriveled biceps, pecs, deltoids, traps, triceps, and, of course, the abs left a long time ago. This physical posturing sets them up for a rounded or kyphotic upper back, a pelvis that is tucked under like a defeated dog, and a head tilted forward with eyes cast to the ground. They look as if they are sad, depressed, defeated, weak, and physically distorted.

Our postures feed back to the brain and release chemicals that help determine how we feel. So holding this defeated posture only triggers more negative and depressed thoughts. Try it in yourself with different postures. Hold the posture described above for one minute, and sense how you feel. My bet is that you won't feel joyful, elated, or ready to tackle your day. If you change your posture to a more anatomically correct stance, which is tall spine, tight core, lifted chest, and upright head, your mood will automatically improve.

I'm wondering if there is some secret held by guys with big bellies. Do they have secret greetings with them, compare sizes, or hold clandestine meetings on how to get them bigger? Whatever it is, they seem to be accepting more and more of the masses into their club.

The great news about all of this is that unless your guy is dead, change can happen, and things can get better. But the opposite is also true as well. Unless your guy is dead, change can happen, and things can get worse. Change in the body is always happening; you are never the same, never. You are either improving or getting worse, even if it is only slightly.

When I was growing up in the 1960s in rural Western Pennsylvania, the older gentlemen in our neighborhood and in our church didn't look like the average guy over forty today, to the best of my recollection.

Think back. Review your old family photograph albums. What did the Dads look like? Remember their physiques and what they did? I don't remember the Dads going to gyms, but I do remember them doing physical work, even if they had desk jobs. They managed a lot of their own home improvements, did gardening, went walking, etc. Sure, there was occasionally a guy or two who would have that beer gut look. In fact, in my case, he was my best friend's father, Mr. Affini, a second-generation Italian. He was the nicest Dad in the neighborhood. He loved to cook, especially pasta, but only with him singing at the top of his lungs with the radio playing Italian polkas.

He worked for the water company reading water meters. Back then, a person had to walk on foot all day and manually read the numbers on a meter. I think he logged a lot of miles in a day. After a day's work, he would come home and make a beeline for the refrigerator, open a cold bottle of beer, and down it in three swallows. Then he'd repeat the process.

He always took the neighborhood kids Halloweening, got them building snowmen, or helped with the girls' softball team. Although he had the physical characteristics of a male menopausal person, I can't think that he had the emotional/physiological characteristics. Anyway, he was the only guy I can remember who had a big belly. Boy, things have changed. Our kids and grandkids are going to be hard-pressed trying to remember an older guy who didn't have a big belly.

There is a hormonal component that manifests itself in physical body types. (We'll take an in-depth review of hormonal factors later. This chapter is about the physical manifestations of hormonal imbalances). Due to the hormonal imbalances of the body, fat is laid down in the tissues in certain places. This pattern is pretty much predicable for men. For women, there are several body types with the accompanying fat patterns that can manifest with hormonal imbalances. Briefly visited, here are the body types. These are from the Body Restoration Technique, Eric Berg, D.C. Does any one of these body types look familiar?

BODY TYPES

THYROID

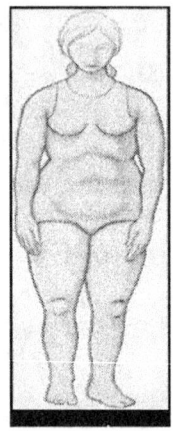

"Butterfly" in the throat area
WEIGHT ALL OVER
Puffiness
Sluggish metabolism
Depressed/apathetic/not motivated
Brain fog/can't complete projects'/the 'messy desk
syndrome'
Craves carbohydrates
Evening fatigue
Hair loss/skin has brown spots/nails are ridged
Cold feet/cold intolerance
Difficulty absorbing vitamins
Decreased sex drive

ADRENAL

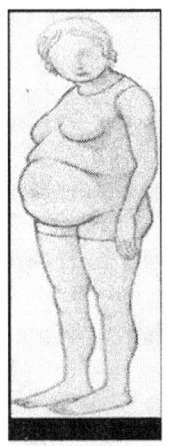

Small organ tissue that sits on top of the kidneys
WEIGHT AROUND THE MIDDLE
Can't sleep well/wakes feeling tired
Winded when climbing stairs
Craves salt and salty foods
'Stressed'/anxiety/worry
Swelling/pain/inflammation
Tight muscles/muscle twitching (potassium loss)

OVARIAN

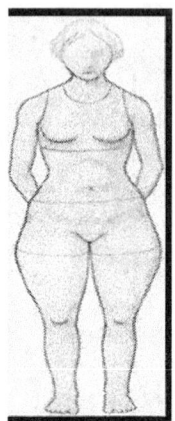

Two inches below and to the side of the navel
SADDLEBAGS AND A LAYER OF FAT BELOW
THE NAVEL
PMS symptoms
Breast tenderness
Menstrual problems
Moodiness
Headache
Bloating and bleeding
Weight gain
Ovarian cysts
Hot flashes
Irritability
Sleeplessness
Vaginal dryness

LIVER

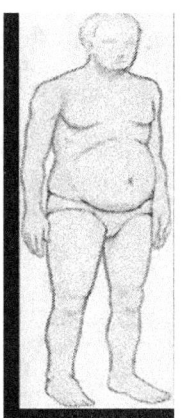

Big organ under the front right rib cage
"BEER BELLY," "POTBELLY," WATER-BELLY
(ascites)
Brown spots on the back of the hands
Yellow eyes
Joint pain/stiffness in the hands, fingers, and back
Right shoulder pain
Cracks on the heels and around the corners of the mouth
Belching and bloating
Difficulty getting out of bed in the morning: morning
grouch who needs coffee
Craves greasy fatty foods

This is just a quick visit to how body types can be correlated with hormonal imbalances. The main thing to remember is that it's not about the physical manifestation of symptoms, such as weight gain, joint aches, weakness, or muscle, fatigue. These, in themselves, are little blessings from your body to tell you that something on the inside is not balanced, that you need help, and that a change is needed. Once the change is made, and the balance is restored inside, these symptoms will vanish. That's how health works!

CHAPTER 5: SEXUAL ISSUES

1. *Less sex drive*

2. *Fewer morning erections*

3. *Erections are not as full*

4. *The size and firmness of the testes are decreased, but the prostate gland size is increased (hypertrophy)*

5. *Less semen*

6. *Weakness on ejaculation with decreased muscle pulsations*

7. *Inability to ejaculate*

8. *All the above can lead to sexual fears and phobias causing a Catch-22.*

Since I am not a guy, I have no firsthand knowledge of male sexual functioning. I don't know how a strong a muscle pulsation versus a weak one would feel to a guy during ejaculation. So I'm going to have to rely on my healthcare background and my research.

There have been so many books written about spicing up your love life with your partner or how to have a more active sex life. Communication, especially if any of these symptoms occur, is very important. Sex is still a taboo subject for some men and woman. Many don't feel comfortable discussing sex or sexual problems, even after decades of marriage and intimacy. If you are in this category, I would suggest getting some recommendations for counselors in your area who work with these issues. A counselor or therapist can be valuable in giving you and your partner a safe space to let your hair down and let it out. And no, it doesn't mean that you're defective or mentally imbalanced because you went to a therapist. It means you care.

Once you and your partner are feeling healthier, more energetic, and have more vitality, your creative juices will be flowing abundantly, and your intimacy and sensuality can only deepen your sexual experience.

Drugs, such as Viagra, and Celledele, have enormous sales annually, so someone must be getting something out of them. In fact, in 2012, annual sales of Viagra pills were over five billion. Five billion! Yikes, that's a lot of pills. While I'm not judging the use of chemical stimulants for increasing sexual pleasure, for purposes of this book, the whole person is considered. That includes many aspects of life, not just sexual function or dysfunction. All drugs have side effects, which are not really side effects; they are effects, even though they are not the desired effects, and they still cause or can cause symptoms that are deleterious, unwanted, and problematic. In a few pages we'll look at common drugs for guys over forty and examine how they may be impacting your guy's life, liberty, and the pursuit of happiness.

CHAPTER 6
HORMONAL/ METABOLIC

What's going on inside?

When there is stuff showing up on the outside, you better believe there is stuff going on in the inside. That's because, just like health and balance, imbalance comes from the inside out. That's how the body works, from the inside out, not the outside in. Thus, we have X-rays, MRI, CT, ultrasound, digital imaging, scoping, stool sampling, and blood work to find internal imbalances before they manifest into the light of day.

In male menopause, the stresses of life, especially mental stress, raise cortisol levels, triggering insulin increases that cause simple carbohydrate cravings and increase the chances of diabetes. The process also makes you fat. There is an imbalance in the fat-storing hormones, which are being produced at a fast rate, and that causes a lowering of the fat-burning hormones. This also affects the testosterone hormone level. This is a key player in male menopause, but it's slightly more complicated than just adding back some testosterone to your body. The amount of estrogen in the male body is also important because it's basically the ratio of testosterone to estrogen that's key. Because certain foods and chemicals have found their way into your guy's body, the natural and normal testosterone-to-estrogen balance has been disturbed. We'll delve into these disruptors within the next few chapters, and we'll look at ways to recognize and avoid them.

So, what exactly is a hormone? A hormone is a body chemical made from cholesterol or protein secreted by an endocrine gland and carried through the blood or lymph system to some other part of the body, where it has a specific effect. An endocrine gland is a gland (tissue) that produces hormones. Examples include thyroid, liver, adrenal, ovary, testicles, and pancreas. There are many hormones in the body. Hormones communicate with your cells. (Can you hear me now!)

In addition, other problems are stirring. These include a worsening of asthma and other breathing issues, kidney and liver problems, light-headedness, dizziness, constipation, varicose veins, high blood pressure, and hemorrhoids, plus a swelling of the ankles due to poor circulation in the legs, and decreased heart muscle mass causing a decrease in the amount of blood that's pumping out of the heart. Trying to pee or urinate becomes increasingly difficult as well. These guys have to go more frequently but have trouble starting the flow, and then it's not a strong flow, maybe a trickle. You've heard the expression, "peeing like a race horse?" Well, this isn't them. Just the opposite.

Just like women, they can experience headaches, hot flashes, heart palpitations, increased heart rate, night sweats, and intolerance to the cold and weather changes. Yikes. With so many problems going on in the body, is it any wonder that they look and act and are so miserable? Let's see what can be done to help solve this problem.

You may think that these symptoms are just part of the normal aging process and unavoidable. Yet studies show[iv] that men have less and less testosterone than their predecessors of just thirty, twenty, or ten years ago. That means that their sons and grandsons will have lower and lower levels as well as time goes on, if nothing is done to counteract this trend.

CHAPTER 7

MAJOR CULPRITS

BEHIND THE CHANGES IN HIS

CHARACTER AND

CHARACTERISTICS

Here are some of the major players in our hormone/metabolic imbalanced dude. Some of these factors within the specific sections are easy to change or modify, while others, depending on your likes or dislikes, can be more of a challenge to address.

DRUGS

Let's start with the drugs he's taking because some of them may be negatively impacting his testosterone levels and actually raising estrogen levels. Remember, as stated before, drugs have side effects, which are actually effects that you may not want. If you want to change or stop medications, I would say to check with the healthcare practitioner who prescribed them. Drugs are powerful substances that cause the physiology of the body to change, and that is why they are prescribed by a professional. But in our culture, the trend is to take a pill first and damn the consequences. Approximately 179,000 people die every year from reactions to properly prescribed drugs and medications.[v] This is not physician error or patient overdose. This is the national statistic for a drug correctly prescribed and correctly taken that resulted in deaths. America spends four trillion dollars on healthcare a year, and yet we are 37th, yes, 37th, in overall health, just below Cuba. So those folks in Cuba stand a better chance of living a longer and healthier life than you and I do. And when it comes to drugs, even though the U.S. population represents under five percent of the world's population, we consume over fifty percent of the world's drugs.[vi] People in other countries don't pop as many pills as we do and seem to be healthier for that fact.

Now it's time to examine drugs. I think you may be surprised at the list:

- *Antidepressants (SSRIs)*
- *Antipsychotics such as Thorazine*
- *Blood thinners, like Coumadin (lots of older folks are on this one.)*
- *Calcium channel blockers like antacids, cimetidine, omeprazole*
- *Anti-convulsants such as phenobarbital, phenytoin*
- *Diuretics*
- *Chemotherapy agents*
- *Antiarrhythmics*
- *Antibiotics*
- *Statins*
- *Antifungal drugs*
- *Propoxyphenes like Darvon*
- *Thyroid suppressing drugs*

- *Opioids like oxycodone are the most-abused prescription drug, and their use and abuse has been rising steadily.[vii]*

- *Marijuana, amphetamines, cocaine, and alcohol*

- *Anti-inflammatory: NSAIDS such as ibuprofen, aspirin, and acetaminophen.*

Looking at this list, how many drugs, whether over-the-counter or prescribed, does the guy in the house eat on a regular basis? The use of NSAIDS, aspirin, and acetaminophen (Advil) is enormous, and they are taken with little regard to the consequences.

ENVIRONMENTAL CHEMICALS:

Okay, who is really tired of trying to keep up with what is environmentally okay these days? Sure, all generations have been exposed to very toxic substances over periods of time. At the time, they seemed safe enough, but in reality they were bad and unhealthy ideas. Think back. Cigarettes, excessive X-rays, thermometers that contained mercury were commonplace. Doctors frequently smoked during patient consultations and treatments. Did you know that it was medical practice to X-ray the baby in the womb to determine its position and size? Or that there were X-ray units in department stores so you could X-ray your feet to see how the shoes fit? Does anyone remember thermometers that contained mercury? They used to break all the time. Just to let you know, mercury is one of the most toxic substances on the planet, and there we were, playing with like it was Play-Doh.

BPAs

A contributor to "old man syndrome" is accumulation of a foreign substance in the body called BPA. This BPA, bisphenol-A, is a chemical used in the production of polycarbonate plastics and epoxy resins. It is prevalent in our environment. It is an estrogen disruptor. According to Wikipedia, "Endocrine disruptors are chemicals that, at certain doses, can interfere with the endocrine (or hormone) system in mammals. These disruptions can cause cancerous tumors, birth defects, and other developmental disorders. Any system in the body controlled by hormones can be derailed by hormone disruptors."

Here's a few ways BPA can be introduced into your environment:

- *Food and drink packaging*
- *Infant bottles*
- *Plastic beverage bottles*
- *Food cans, bottle tops*
- *Water supply pipes*
- *Dental sealant and composites*
- *CDs*
- *Impact-resistant safety devices*
- *Medical devices*

When exposed to heat, this chemical leaches out of the plastic and into you. It causes so many problems in your body and one of the problems is that it makes you fat because it causes estrogen to be made. It's also linked to cancer. Many other countries ban BPA, but it's plentiful here in the U.S.

My husband, a doctor, gave an eye-opening presentation about this chemical a few years back, and since then I haven't drunk out of a plastic bottle or wrapped any hot food into anything plastic. We replaced plastic containers with glass and have stainless-steel, glass, or BPA-free water bottles, and buy only BPA-free canned goods. You can do an Internet search for BPA-free brands of canned food products. Recently both Del Monte and Campbell's soup products have changed to BPA free lined cans. Here is a short synopsis how to curtail your exposure to BPA:

- *Avoid plastic containers for food and drinks*
- *Never put plastic in the microwave*
- *Try to buy only BPA-free cans*
- *Use stainless steel, glass, wood, or ceramic instead of plastic for storage containers, cookware, and spoons*
- *No plastic wrap on hot food*

The plastic is pandemic and insidious. We live with plastic all around us all the time. While preparing a health talk on the evils of BPA, especially how heat and plastic don't mix, I was making myself a cup of coffee from our recent splurge on a new coffee maker that makes just one cup. You stick the little plastic container of coffee in the machine, push the start button, and steaming hot water passes through the plastic, and out comes your coffee. What? It dawns on me! Heat and plastic don't mix. I said a sad good-bye to my fancy coffee maker and then realized that most coffee makers have plastic tubing that the hot water runs through. Go check yours. I bet there is plastic. So now we use the old-fashioned stainless-steel electric percolators. Again, BPA is an estrogen disruptor and contributes to many health issues.

How prevalent is BPA? The CDC (Centers for Disease Control) tested 2,517 urine samples,[viii] which is a sizable study. Subjects were six years and older. The study revealed that 93 per cent tested positive for detectable levels of BPA. THINK!!!

Two groups of rats were fed the exact same diet. One group was exposed to low levels of BPA (*Endocrinology* 2011 August 152(8)). The group that was exposed to the BPA became obese. There is an informative article written by Brian Bienkowski, (*Environmental Health News*, Sept. 18 2012). Another interesting read is *Our Stolen Future* by Colbon, Dumanoski, and Myers.

ARTIFICIAL HORMONES

Among the other chemicals that cause both obesity and cancer because, once again, they are estrogen disruptors, are artificial hormones. These are added to animal feed and injected into animals, and when we eat the animals or products that come from them, we eat the hormonal residue. Yuck! This has been linked to girls reaching puberty at an earlier age, the feminization of men, cancer, and obesity.[ix] In the early 1990s, European nations banned the importing of American meat because of the hormones and other chemicals in our animals. Why is it that other countries seem to be more stringent about the chemicals and products that they allow in the food sources and the chemicals that they use?

The things you can do about decreasing your artificial hormone ingestion are very simple but will cost you more money in the short run. Buy organic meat and animal products. I am so thankful that there is such a thing as organic animal products.

I don't eat meat and haven't for the past forty years, but I do eat cheese, a little milk, and rarely butter. When purchasing these products, I really try to buy organic and hormone-free. Even eggs can be purchased from chickens that aren't fed hormones. Oh, by the way, I don't push my way of eating on anybody. I did that in the first decade I was vegetarian, only to alienate myself and piss off a lot of people. My in-laws in particular.

After fifteen years of being a vegetarian, I met a great guy in graduate school. He was from Montana, a farm kid, as he likes to say.

If you know anything about Montana, you know that it largely concerns cattle ranching and hunting. He should have had two strikes against him. But love never knows about the "shoulds." You know what I mean. My husband and I fell hard in love with each other, even though our worlds were far apart. We met in chiropractic college, I in my early 30s and he in his mid-30s. I had never been married and never wanted to marry. He had been married for twelve years, had two boys, and had been divorced for three years. I had lived in many states and traveled to many countries. I was a vegetarian who explored many different dietary regimes, including macrobiotics and raw foods diets. I liked Tai chi and yoga and avant-garde dress. He hadn't been out of Montana; had no other pants than blue jeans, ate two-for-a-dollar hot dogs, mostly purchased at gas stations; had hunted; and had come from a cattle ranching/farming family. Could two people be so seemingly opposite? But despite these outward differences, we fell in love and married. When he introduced me to his family and announced that he too was not eating meat any more, his family, especially his mother thought that he had married the devil demon herself. I stood for everything she thought was weird, and she told him, "There is nothing good about that girl." Sometimes one just needs a few decades of time and hanging around to change someone's opinion, and that's exactly what I did. I got a lot less preachy about the meat thing, and they all got a lot more accepting of me and my life choices. I think we all were better for it.

I guess the lesson here is that when you make changes in your diet and the foods you eat, you may get a lot of flak and lip from your family and friends. Be true to what you want, thank them for their opinion and input, and go on with your life.

GMOs

There is one more item I'd like to include in the "please, please, please" avoid category. This one is pretty difficult to avoid if you are living in the United States, and there is not much evidence of any harm that it's doing as of yet. But, again, many countries in the world are not allowing GMOs, or genetically modified organisms. And they are requiring food labeling of GMO products. Go and research GMOs, and you'll see for yourself what the buzz is about.

Recently, the wonderful and talented Neil Young came to my town for a concert. During the concert he mentioned his disdain for GMOs. I thought it was wonderful. However, I was very surprised at the number of people who had never heard of GMOs and had no idea what he was talking about.

GMOs are created when an organism has been altered by having its DNA changed by inserting DNA that has been modified or engineered to produce a particular result. The DNA can be laboratory-made, come from another organism, or come from the same organism.

There are four major food crops that are GMO, and they are corn, soybeans, canola, and sugar beets. You may think you don't eat sugar beets, but most sugar beets are grown for sugar. So if you eat sugar or products that contain sugar, they probably come from GMO foods. Soy, soy lecithin, and most soy products are GMO. Many people think that wheat is GMO but a significant portion of the U.S. wheat crop is exported. Since other countries ban GMOs, our wheat would not be able to be purchased by other countries if it were GMO.

The non-profit organization, Non-GMO Project, provides third-party testing to assure manufacturers that their products are non-GMO. Look for their logo/label on products.

Now that your curiosity and interest in GMOs has been sparked, do a little research on your own to ascertain your own knowledge and opinion about whether you want to continue ingesting food that is made with GMOs.

The other thing you can do to avoid GMO is buy organic! Organic food, to be labeled as such, cannot contain GMOs. Presently, I know of no research that links GMO foods with obesity, increased estrogen, or decreased testosterone. But when you start looking into GMOs, it's just too spooky, like a science-fiction horror story. That's just my opinion. I suggest you do a little or a lot of research and investigation on your own and make up your own mind. Until you do, I'd definitely recommend buying organic and bypassing those sugar beets!

The "cleaner" and less toxic your body can become on a cellular level, the healthier you will be and the better you will feel.

CHAPTER 8
THREE PHASES TO A FUNNER
BUDDY

Now on to the program that can potentially transform that chubby and cranky thing on your couch into a being with more of a resemblance to that guy that you hooked up with in the first place. Keep in mind that this is a process, and there is no process that doesn't take time and effort. How much time and how much effort is up to you. What you put in, you will get out. You will get frustrated and maybe give up for a time. It's natural and human nature. The important part is that you begin again. Keep at it. And if you do backslide or if he backslides, don't go crazy with guilt and shame. Just start again. That's usually how change, long-term change, is accomplished.

Oops, I just said a nasty and scary word. Change! I know; you hate it. My joke to myself when asked to change is, "I changed once; I didn't like it. I'm not doing that again!"

As a primary-care physician, I get so frustrated with the mantra of health: Eat right and exercise. Physicians are constantly telling their patients to exercise. I disagree. True, the joints in the body need to move in all directions every day to get rid of metabolic waste products and get fresh nutrients for joint health. And I truly think exercise is essential to feeling and functioning well.

Exercise can help lower blood sugar levels, decrease blood pressure, improve sleep, improve cardiovascular health, and increase testosterone levels.

However, to tell an obese patient who is in continual pain, feeling very unhealthy, and hasn't done a thing in years, to "go exercise" is not helpful, in my eyes. Many people have confided in me, over the years, their frustration with being told by their primary care physicians during a physical examination to eat right and exercise. They don't know where to begin or how. The patients first need to get to a baseline health level, and then they can make nutritional and exercise changes that will jump-start their program.

There are three phases of this program, therefore, and each phase has three essential components that need to be addressed and followed:

1. **Food:** what you put into your mouth
2. **Supplements:** something extra to heal, repair, and maintain your wonderful cells and tissues
3. **Exercise:** what you do to increase strength, flexibility, balance, cardiovascular health, and happiness

PHASE I

In this phase of the program, it will look like not much of anything is happening, at least from the outside, but inside healing is happening. Your life is changing for the better!

FOOD

You can make most of the same foods and meals that you would normally make, only you are going to start buying only organic meat, animal products, vegetables, fruits, breads, grains, even desserts and snacks. You are now an organic kitchen! There is one little thing to be aware of here. Sticker shock. Yep, using less-expensive chemicals, dyes, and pesticides on your grocery items means a bigger bill at the checkout stand. I never really understood that, but it's been evident since I started purchasing organic foods thirty years ago. If you have a farmer's market in your area, explore your organic options there first because it may be less expensive.

One arena worth addressing here is the eating out in restaurants and fast-food joints. I cannot stress enough that fast-food joints are not the best places to eat; in fact, they may be close to the bottom, next to gas station vending machines. You know this. Everyone older than five years old knows this. Yet every time I drive past one of them, there is a line of cars. The "burger heads," we call them. Wait; Maybe they are all getting salads! During this phase, try your best not to eat out. Look, you know tomorrow about noon you are probably going to get hungry. It's not going to be a surprise. So be prepared by packing a lunch beforehand. It's that easy. Save the eating out to times when it may be required of you because of a business lunch or other occasion.

In addition to eating organic, and eating in, there is one other slight change in this phase concerning intake, and that is beverages. If you drink soda pop or energy drinks, stop. Period. Drink water. And don't think that because you drink a diet pop, you are exempt. Drink water. I tell patients that I'd rather they drink vodka than diet sodas, because the vodka is better for them. Of course, I really wasn't condoning it or encouraging them to drink vodka; it was to educate them on how potentially bad diet sodas are, health-wise. They make you bloat and swell, have no nutritional value, and are full of chemicals and potential neurotoxins. None for you! Drink water.

IT'S SUPPLEMENT TIME

You are going to set out to find the least-expensive and best-quality supplements and nutritional products. Put those by his breakfast and make sure he swallows them. It's been my experience that guys don't know what pills they're taking, generally speaking. If you put it out and say take it, it will be down the hatch. If he asks what it is, you don't need to lie, say it's something to help them feel and look better. Vague is usually a good tack to take.

Here is a list of supplements to start with. These nutritional products ought not to interfere with medications, but I'd suggest checking their compatibility with any drugs or medications that are being taken with your doctor or pharmacist. While there are some supplements you both can take, you will not want to take his, and he won't want to take yours.

Both: Omega-3 fatty acids. This is also known as fish oil. It can be taken in pill or liquid form. Recommendations vary, though the most popular thought is 2500 to 3500mg/day. This is taken to help with inflammation, circulation, and brain functioning. Do you think you and hubby could use this?

Both: Multivitamin/mineral supplement. My research has convinced me that you likely aren't getting all your necessary nutrition from your food. The Dietary Reference Intakes (DRIs) are developed and published by the Institute of Medicine (IOM). The DRIs represent the nutrient needs of most average and healthy people.

Here is a very useful link for DRIs:

https://fnic.nal.usda.gov/sites/fnic.nal.usda.gov/files/up loads/recommended_intakes_individuals.pdf

In order for you to get adequate DRIs the USDA has a user-friendly picture that you can find on-line or in public school cafeterias. In 2011 the USDA replaced the food pyramid with MyPlate. In all meals, one half of your plate ought to consist of fruits and vegetables, the other half protein and grains, with a saucer size of dairy on the side. This represents approximately nine servings of fruits and vegetables daily, which is the recommendation from the Department of Health and Human Services.

Does your plate look like this every meal? Are you getting nine servings of fruits and veggies daily? Doubtful. This is one reason for vitamin and mineral supplementation.

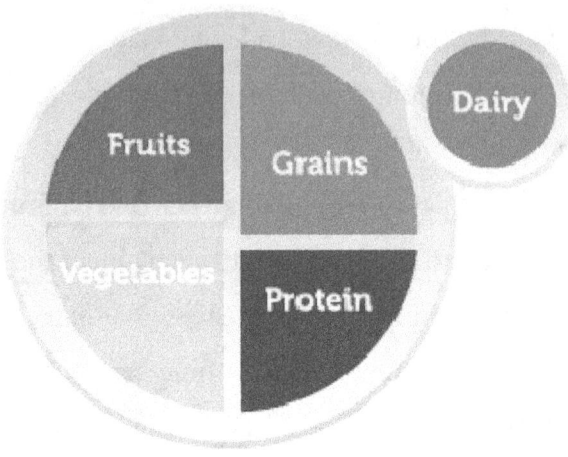

Unless you're the exception, take the vitamin. Pure Encapsulations out of Massachusetts has balanced formulas for him and her. (I don't benefit from recommending this particular nutritional company. There are many good ones.)

For him: Also from Pure Encapsulations is something called Tribulus Formula. This is a combination of vitamins and herbs to help the body maintain normal testosterone levels.

You know, the main thing about these supplements, aside from purchasing them, is that you have to actually put them in your mouth and swallow them. I know it sounds simple, but just because you buy them doesn't mean they're helping you. You have to actually put them in your mouth and swallow them. Many patients of mine, when asked if they are taking such and such vitamin, say, "Well, I have it because I bought it, but I forgot to take it." It's important, so do it.

The trick is to add nutrients that will help the body increase testosterone levels, and this is a balancing act. It works like your checkbook. If you spend more than you deposit, you are going to have a deficiency. So, while you're increasing your testosterone levels, you want to do things that will not cause a decrease in the levels. Thus, no BPAs, and no artificial hormones that are added to non-organic meat and dairy products. Another item to avoid is soy, as in soybeans, tofu, or soy sauce just to name a few. Ladies, you may be familiar with soy as a supplement you would take to increase your estrogen, especially during menopause. The guys don't want the estrogen, so no soy for them. Again, be sure the soy that is used in your house is organic. Ninety-four percent of the soy grown in the U.S. is GMO, according to the USDA Department of Agriculture.

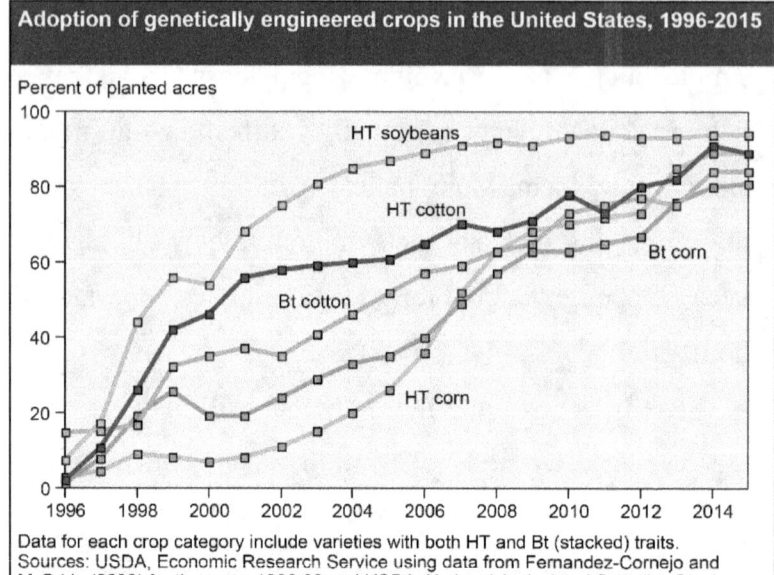

Adoption of genetically engineered crops in the United States, 1996-2015

Percent of planted acres

Data for each crop category include varieties with both HT and Bt (stacked) traits.
Sources: USDA, Economic Research Service using data from Fernandez-Cornejo and
McBride (2002) for the years 1996-99 and USDA, National Agricultural Statistics Service,
June Agricultural Survey for the years 2000-15.

PLANTING THE "WORKOUT" SEED

As I stated previously, at this stage in the game, I wouldn't recommend an exercise program, per se. Too many times, people, especially guys, will want to start where they left off forty years ago. So they'll hit the gym and be disappointed and/or physically damaged because they couldn't lift the same weight they did in their twenties, or they can't run as far or as fast as they did when they ran track in high school. Exercise ought not to be about failure but about fun. So, at this point, just plant the seed that exercise, fun exercise, will be in his future.

You can discuss what types of exercise or activity you'd both like to do. And it doesn't have to be the same. Let your mind drift back to when you were young. What sorts of activities did you enjoy, and how can you extrapolate that into an appropriate exercise activity now?

For example, one of my youngest and most treasured memory is pretending to be a ballerina. On Saturday nights my sisters and I would don our petticoats and dance while my mother played classic pieces on the piano. Later, I found baton twirling. I loved being a majorette in junior high school. I would listen to records and make routines up to the songs, mostly marches, and twirl that baton in all kinds of moves and directions. Then I'd march up and down the street with some song going in my head, along with my two sisters, also majorettes. Yes, the neighbors thought my parents put something goofy in our food.

Today, forty-five years later, my passionate exercise is OULA, which is a high-octane dance fitness. After a class, which is about an hour, I'm a sweaty mess with a big smile. I love it and can't wait to do it as often as possible. I even got certified to teach it.

It may take some introspection to find what you use to love to do and create your new version of what that may look like. Most children loved some form of activity. Think back. What was yours? How can you modify or re-tool that activity to transform it into an exercise that fits your current lifestyle?

I always get asked by patients, "What is the best exercise to do?" I say, "The one that you love to do and are passionate about because that is the one that you will stick with, in the long run." If I say swimming is the best exercise, and you hate the water, then you're not going to do that program. This is another way people set themselves up for workout failure.

Another failure feature is the buddy system. Unless your activity involves something like scuba diving, you don't always need a buddy. It's too easy for the buddy to lose motivation and drop out, giving you the perfect reason to stop your workouts. Many personal trainers recommend the buddy system as a motivational technique, but I think that too many times it also can be an excuse to quit. But, it really depends on your motivational style. If you are intrinsically or internally motivated, you don't need external nudging, like prizes for workouts completed or a workout buddy to keep you motivated. However, if you are in the external motivation camp, you are going to have to make your exercise routine interesting and fun. A motivational buddy may be the ticket to hold you accountable.

SUMMARY FOR PHASE 1

- Buy organic.
- Eat out less, especially avoiding fast-food establishments.
- Make your own lunches in advance.
- Buy a glass or stainless-steel water bottle and ditch those plastic bottles.
- Replace plastic food containers with glass.
- Get the recommended supplements, and eat them daily.
- Think about what type of exercise you'd love to start doing.

TIME FRAME

So how long should you do PHASE 1? That is up to you. You start with where you are right now. If you already are doing some or all of these things, then with a little fine-tuning, things can turn around in as quickly as two weeks. If this is all foreign to you, and you and hubby are looking, feeling, and functioning pretty poorly, then I suggest at least one to two months for this transition. After that time, you will feel and see a significant change in your body and your mental outlook. You are going to feel and function so much better.

CHAPTER 9

PHASE II

From now on things are going to get much easier. The difficult part is behind you. You did it!

Now, we are going to refine your diet a bit more, continue your supplements, and start an exercise program. If you backslide a little due to a change in your routine, holiday seasons, parties, or vacations, that's okay. It's called being human. The main thing is that you get back on the horse and start again.

DIET

Did you know that the common denominator of successful dietary change and sustained weight loss is keeping track of what you eat? It is termed a diet diary. Studies from the University of Pittsburgh Diabetes Prevention Support Center and Kaiser Permanente's Center for Health Research have found that people who kept a daily diet diaries lost twice as much weight as those who didn't keep daily food records. A diet diary is a sure way to be conscious about exactly what you are eating. You can do this several ways. For three days (it's only three days), write down what foods and how much of them you ate. Then go online or look at the package to determine the amount of calories you ate in that day. For instance, if the package says twelve corn chips are one-hundred-and-fifty calories, then take twelve from the bag or multiples of that. While I don't think it's feasible to measure everything you eat for life, this exercise is extremely powerful and a real eye-opener. After the three days, you can either write down what you ate, or, if you are pretty aware of your eating habits, you can just remember and go through a mental list. The problem with the latter method, the one you do only in your head, is that you will inevitably forget those things that you don't want to remember, like the candy bar, scone, or bag of potato chips. So, at least in the beginning, and to keep you honest with yourself, write it down.

In the beginning of this phase, this is all you need to do. Keep a diet diary and calorie count for three days, and then a written diary of what you ate for two weeks.

SUPPLEMENTS

Supplements are going to stay the same as in the initial phase. Don't forget to write them down as something you consume. This will also insure that you are actually taking them on a daily basis.

EXERCISE

This is where you start to move that body. Exercise is so misunderstood in our culture. Maybe because, overall, we as a nation are very sedentary and also very overweight. Sixty percent of the US population is now overweight, according to the new CDC statistics. (http://www.cdc.gov/ obesity/resources/index.html). When I ask patients if they exercise, many times I hear the answer, "Well, I try to walk." Bingo! When someone says they try to exercise, I know that they are not exercising, only wishing to "try." Walking is a great place to start exercising, providing that you have a safe place to walk, great weather to walk in, and don't have bad hips, knees, ankles or feet. I live in Montana, where open space and parks are plentiful. It's a great place to walk and very dog-friendly. Research has shown that having a dog that needs walking daily is great incentive for people to get out and exercise.[x] However, the problem is that it gets really cold here in Montana for a large portion of the year. It also is dark a large portion of the day throughout the winter. So, if I don't want to walk in the frigid temperatures, ice, and dark I'm probably going to nix my walking as exercise program pretty quickly. That's why it is so important to find something that you love and will do every day. What? Did I just mention exercise daily? OK, well most days, at least. The American Council of Exercise recommends at least 150 minutes of moderate to vigorous exercise per week. That's at least 2.5 hours of real workout time per week. Moderate to vigorous doesn't include casual strolls or running around the office. It is sustained accelerated heart rate.

Guess what is the number one perceived barrier to exercise? TIME! Actually it is thinking that there is not enough time to include exercise in our busy days. But, guess how many hours Americans average in front of the TV per week? Approximately twenty-two hours, according to the United States Department of Labor, Bureau of Labor Statistics. And according to The Statista, Americans view thirty-three hours of television weekly. Interesting statistics.

I'm not encouraging everyone to join a gym and become a "gym rat." There are plenty of workouts you can do in your home that require very little space and few items of equipment. A yoga mat, tubing, some free weights, a few videos, and you are good to go. Again, you may have a whole gym in your basement with shelves full of fabulous workout CDs and a big screen TV, but you just aren't motivated to exercise. This is where, initially, a buddy may come in handy. Invite them to join you. Make it fun. Schedule your workouts as if they were written in stone. And, again, make it fun so you will eventually look forward to it and be sad if you miss your workout.

Growing up in northern Pennsylvania, it was fairly cold in the autumn and that lasted until May. It also got dark about five p.m. in the afternoon. My father was usually in pretty good shape, even though he had a sedentary job as an engineer. There were six of us living in a small three-bedroom one-bath house, and there wasn't much room. I remember that when it was winter, and he couldn't play golf, do yard work, or another outside activity, he would use a small area in my parents' bedroom, maybe four feet by six feet, and do exercises that he got out of a military exercise book. He'd jog in place, and do jumping jacks, sit-ups, and other exercises. He didn't do them for long, maybe half-an-hour, and he didn't do them every day, maybe three to four times per week. But he did them every week. That is the key. Consistency. Don't think you need to spend hours daily exercising. You'll probably last a total of three days. Do what you can when you can, and be consistent.

Now that you've thought about what you loved to do as a child and have extrapolated that to some exercise program you'd like to start, I'd like you to shuffle back to page 21 to examine the hormone body types. Don't study them; just ask yourself which one you are and go with your initial impression. I know if I look at the types long enough, I can see myself in every one. But there is one that I initially thought, "Ah, that's me!"

If you fit into the thyroid or liver hormone type, your exercise will aim to be more anaerobic. Anaerobic exercise does not require as much oxygen to be delivered to the muscles. Types of Anaerobic exercise include sprinting and weight lifting. If you fit into the adrenal or ovary hormone type, your exercise will be slanted to aerobic activities. Aerobic exercise requires the use of oxygen carried to the muscles. Common types of aerobic exercise include running, dancing, swimming, and biking.

But please don't get too hung up on the type of exercise. Just do something to start. Too many times, procrastinators overanalyze something and end up doing nothing. So don't overthink this by studying how many repetitions and sets of each exercise should be done in lieu of actually doing the exercise. The healthier you become, the more your own innate intelligence will shine through, and you will innately know what types of activities you should engage in and for how long and for how many times per week.

I have a friend, Donald, who now is in his early sixties, but yearns to be in the shape he was in when he was twenty-five. Not unusual. So he hired a personal trainer at his local gym and had a thorough consult before he started his training regime. Donald and most of us over fifty-five (I guess that constitutes senior citizens) have had a few too many accidents, injuries, and the like from our youthful sports frolics and other daredevil accidents, not to mention the garden variety auto accidents, bicycling accidents, hard work, etc. It's been several months, and Donald is still at it, working out in the gym multiple times per week, sometimes with the help of his trainer. This is such a smart thing to do. Congratulations, Donald; keep up the great work. Good health doesn't cost; it pays.

Jack on the other hand is a very stubborn guy when it comes to his exercise regime. He thinks he is an expert because twenty years ago he spent some time in a gym with a guy who knew how to "work out." Jack constantly is hurting himself in the gym because he has poor form and won't ask for help. So after he injures his shoulder, knee, hip, or other body part, he can't and won't go back for months. Then he'll try to do the same routine he did previous to his last injury, which causes him to re-injure the body part, and the cycle continues.

It only takes two weeks for you to become de-conditioned. I know; it's totally unfair. But if you take time off from exercise, start easy and work your way up again.

TO RECAP PHASE II

Your diet is about the same as in PHASE I, with more structure. You're keeping a diet diary or diet log, and for at least three to seven days, you specifically figure out the calories in your food. You may even want to log the percentage of carbohydrates, proteins, and fats in your diet diary/food log. Supplements are the same, and be consistent! This is the part where you may have run out of your supplements, finishing your first bottle. Go get more; don't go without them.

Many times patients would stop taking their nutritional supplements, and when I asked them why, they would say they didn't feel much difference with them. At this point, I would whack them over the head with their chart and show them what they said on specific dates. "Argh, Ms. Jones, do you see my chart notes from four weeks ago? I'll read what it says: "Ms. Jones claims to be sleeping much better throughout the night and has increased energy throughout the day since starting on supplements. Also, pain levels are reduced, gone from eight to five." "Well, I guess the supplements were helping after all. I'll get more and start back on them." It's not just Ms. Jones. I've seen this so many times. We as humans forget quickly, especially if it is about ourselves. It's like we need someone to hold up a mirror so we can honestly see and reflect about ourselves and our lives. So, bottom line, take your supplements.

The biggest change in this phase concerns your exercise regime because now you are initiating and actually performing regular exercise. Woohoo! Good for you, and keep it up when little interruptions such as life get in your way.

By now your kitchen is looking a little different. Right? There are no more inorganic foods and there may be no GMO foods. There are no plastic water bottles and no plastic containers, no plastic spoons or forks. You now let food cool completely before even waving anything plastic at it, like plastic wrap, plastic bags, or plastic anything.

You may have all your supplements out on the countertop just to remind yourself to give them to hubby or take them yourself. You are finding that the money that you spent eating out and ordering sodas or fatty coffee drinks is better spent on your whole organic foods and dietary supplements.

Because your taste buds are changing for the better, your pantry has a lot less crap food, such as processed sugary items and salty greasy snack foods. Your refrigerator is stocked full of veggies and fruits and healthier organic foods, which you are now learning to cook.

Cooking whole foods is much different than microwaving a prepackaged food item isn't it? It takes time for the preparation, and, let's face it, there are mistakes that have been made and that will continue to be made. I'm with you. I've ruined so many potentially delicious dishes. One of my problems is that I have a hard time following a recipe. It should be easy enough for someone who has a nutrition degree plus a doctorate, but something often goes awry with my cooking.

It was my first dinner gathering, and I was jinxed from the start. When I was eighteen, a friend and I were making dinner at her new apartment. We had invited two really cute boys over, hoping to entice them to like us by cooking a wonderful dinner. We were both vegetarians, which they knew, and had recently discovered Francis Moore Lappe's cookbook, *Diet for a New Planet*. This fabulous groundbreaking cookbook had all kinds of foods which we were unfamiliar to me. So Annie and I decided to dive in and experiment with these foods. Like beans that weren't from a can, just dried beans.

Well, I forgot to do one little thing with those raw beans I cooked. I must have skipped the line that said "soak the beans overnight." The dish resembled eating bullets, not beans. We still had a lot of fun, and luckily the guys were smart enough to stop and eat before they came, just in case. My friend now owns a restaurant and is the chief chef. She continues to cook delicious and creative dishes. Me, not so much.

My most recent effort was my tenth attempt at making homemade gnocchi. On our trip to Italy, I was amazed at this food. I had had the little potato balls as a child. My mother served them, but they were always something that came in a bag, not homemade. In Italy, the gnocchi were light, like little fluffy potato pillows. My last attempt didn't turn out any better than the previous nine, only this time I was serving it at a dinner party and it was pretty much the main course. I asked my brave husband to taste one. He gallantly popped one in his mouth, made a grotesque face, spit the gnocchi ball out, and announced, "Honey, I can choke down just about anything, but I can't eat this." I quickly made something else and tried to save the remainder of the gnocchi fiasco. I got creative and made it into a casserole-looking thing. When dinner came and all food was on the table and we were all happily eating, someone spotted the gnocchi fiasco casserole thing. With total surprise and wide eyes, they gasped, "What's that?" pointing to my dish of embarrassment. "Oh, that," I said, "It's a new recipe from my wonderful Italian cookbook. It's called Fecola Patate."

Well, some tried the Fecola Patate, but in the end we threw most of it out. We did learn something from the Fecola Patate experience. If something goes wrong with a dish, just re-invent it some way and look in your cookbooks to find a name that sounds delicious and exotic, call it that and watch folks try it. Hey, it worked with my husband's last birthday cake that turned out to be more like a gel. I served it up as "Italian Hazelnut Bombay." I made him an organic box cake as well, and threw most of the Bombay in the garbage. Now go make your own mistakes.

SUMMARY FOR PHASE II

- **Diet** continues as in PHASE I
- **Supplements** continue as in PHASE I

- **Exercise** for at least two and one-half hours weekly and be sure it is moderate to vigorous.

TIME FRAME

Enjoy this exciting time, when you and partner are looking and feeling much better. You're making better and better choices and seeing results. This time period can last between one to six months. Though I bet after one month you will tire of keeping your diet diary. Just keep at it.

CHAPTER 10

PHASE III

Okay, this is it. This is your new and improved life, and you will want to continue on this regime for life. But before you start crying because you will never be able to have another hot fudge sundae or a container of Pringles, stop. Don't be ridiculous. You are here to enjoy food, friends, and family, among other things. So go for it, just not every day. At this point, you are healthy enough to occasionally binge on something that used to be a favorite. I'm going to wager that, while it's going in the mouth and down the food tube, it's going to feel heavenly, but you may not feel that good the next day.

It's like me and Coca-Cola. Growing up, I would pour big glasses of the stuff, grab a red licorice stick, chew off the ends, and use it as a straw to suck down the vat of Coca-Cola.   Yep, that was a lot of sugar and chemicals. Now, about twice a year, usually when I'm on a long plane trip, the flight attendant will ask if I want something to drink, and I'll surprise myself by saying, "Coke, please." It tastes so good. I say, "Man, I know why people buy these and drink them by the six-packs." But after the fourth sip, I'm done. It just tastes too weird for me, like those yellow marshmallow Peeps at Easter or those wax lips at Halloween. All are in the yucky category. But a couple of times a year, I need to be reminded. Enjoy, or not, those foods and drinks that you would have killed for, with much discretion.

DIET

It's time to experiment! Yeah, I love experimenting on myself with food and diet. I want you to notice how eating certain foods or nutrients makes you feel, physically, mentally, and emotionally. And yes, food does affect your emotions and your ability to think clearly. How you find out the effect of a food or nutrient is to pretty much eliminate that particular food or food item from your diet for a period of time, usually ten days is recommended. Then add it back or load it, and load a lot of it and see what it does to you. It's possible that you may see no change or you may see drastic and dramatic changes in your health.

Here are a few food items that a significant part of the population is sensitive to:

Gluten: This is the protein in wheat. The elimination of gluten tends to be difficult for people, and I never suggest it lightly to patients. We eat so much wheat, and the wheat seeds have been hybridized so as to not even resemble the wheat seeds that your grandparents and great-grandparents knew. Gluten is in breads, pastas, cookies, pastries, crackers, and cakes. You can substitute rice flour, garbanzo flour, and coconut flour just to name a few. There are plenty of gluten-free items available now, all at an increased fee over the gluten products. I even saw a fast-food pizza chain down the road advertise that they have gluten free pizza. Be careful, though; there are a couple of items used in gluten-free products that ought to be avoided. These are tapioca flour (very fattening), potato starch, and cornstarch. A wonderful and easy-to-read book delving into this subject is *Wheat Belly: Lose the Wheat, Lose the*

Weight, and Find Your Path Back to Health by William Davis, M.D. He's a cardiologist out of the Midwest. In his book, Davis recounts his research into the changes in the type of wheat that is presently grown as compared to the days of our grandparents. It is his opinion that the big bellies seen on so many Americans are from over-consumption of wheat. It's an easy and good read. I'd suggest this eye-opening book.

Dairy: Did someone say pass the butter? No…no, I love cheese. I could do without all the other dairy and animal foods, but I do love cheese. Sometime back, I did a strict macrobiotic diet, which was void of dairy, along with many other foods. After five years, a friend from Southern California made some amazing-looking thing called nachos. I politely ate one, even though it was covered in cheese. That was it. It's cheeseaholic time! Dairy includes milk, cheese, and butter. Actually, now I go through periodic abstention from dairy and always feel better in my joints and sinuses. Give it a try!

Soy: If you think soy is that stuff tofu is made from, you're correct. And soy is in just about everything these days. You are going to need to read labels, so don't forget your reading glasses when grocery shopping. Look for the ingredients soy and soy lecithin. Soy lecithin is a lipid-type substance (phospholipid) that is used to emulsify or break down chunky types of fat to small molecules. In the food industry, it is used to coat chocolate and to make liquids and semi-solid foods, such as salad dressings and sauces, creamier and have a better consistency, and it is in everything from ice cream, to bread, to candy bars, to protein drinks.

Elizabeth, a wonderful woman I know, told me about her soy-sensitivity discovery. Most mornings, she would do a protein drink containing soy. A couple of hours later, she would "crash" both physically and mentally. Plus, she would get emotionally depressed. Knowing this wasn't her normal energetic and cheery self, she began a dietary self-exploration that led her to the culprit, soy. As long as she avoids it, she feels really good.

Sugar: Oh no, I said the "S" word. This item, sugar, is also in many food items that you would not suspect, like ketchup, tomato sauce, and salad dressing. Again, read the labels if you're buying processed and packaged food and remember your reading glasses, you're going to need them because the print is often very small. The American Heart Association recommends that women should have no more than 100 calories/day of added sugar and guys 150 calories. And that is all forms of sugar, including corn syrup and high fructose corn syrup.

I remember reading a book in the 1980s called *Sugar Blues* by William Duffy. It was a major eye-opener. If you can get hold of a copy, read it just to get a little historical background. At the turn of the last century, the average American ate one pound of sugar per year. Now it's increased to one-hundred-and-thirteen pounds/year/person. Oh no! So, try to cut down or totally eliminate sugar from your diet and notice the difference it makes in your weight, energy level, mood, emotions, etc.

Why does it happen that someone can eat a particular food their entire life and suddenly begin to react to that food? I've seen that happen many times, and I'm sure practicing allergists and immunologists will agree. Someone can eat nuts galore all their life and suddenly start to have allergic reactions of hives, dermatitis, and other symptoms. Is it because the body has hit a threshold of tolerance and beyond that point it will not be balanced, like the tipping point? Is it that the food item itself has a different quality about it, such as hybrid plants or genetically modified seeds? Or is it that the intestinal wall gets irritated and becomes more porous, allowing larger molecules into the body and thus into the bloodstream? The body sees these larger molecules in the blood as bad and foreign things, things that need attacking, and so to defend itself, the body attacks these things, which actually are itself. So the body attacks itself because it's confused. The result is that you feel poorly but can't quite figure out what/s going on. This brief description of a rather complex situation is called "Leaky Gut Syndrome." What a name! It makes me think I need a little Dutch boy to plug the leaks in my intestines.

While the mechanism of action, that is the "why" of the situation, is not clear, avoidance of the reactive food substances will make you feel so much better. I think that a food sensitivity can be changed, and, after a long period of doing without, one could be able to tolerate a small dose of the offending item once in a while. But this is something you are going to need to experiment with on your own.

Throughout my thirty years of being on the nutrition radar, I have seen so many dietary regimes come and go. These are termed fad diets. Fad diets are usually marketed to be fast, easy, and have the famous "they" recommending the newest diet. Who are "they," and why do "they" think "they" know what is best for me when it comes to what I put in my mouth for nourishment?

We are as different on the inside as we are on the outside, and thus we all have different needs when it comes to our diet and exercise. Throughout my thirty years of researching, writing, and counseling patients about diet and nutrition, however, their predominant focus always seems to be on the latest trend or food fad. They included the grapefruit diet, fen-phen diet, all-protein diet, macrobiotic diet, raw-food diet, eat right for your type diet, Atkins diet, and the HCG diet. I'm sure I've forgotten a few dozen.

In the diet/nutrition quagmire of information, we are laying some scientific and physiologic building blocks about the body and its nutritional and energy needs. Let's look at some ideas to help you identify the food choices and eating patterns that will allow your best and healthiest self to shine.

I grew up in Middle America circa the 1960s with meat, potatoes, canned vegetables, and sugar. It was all pretty processed, like Velveeta cheese, hot dogs, canned peas, and doughnuts. Breakfast was sugared cereal with artificial colors, lunch in the school cafeteria was mystery meat with white bread, and dinner was mac and cheese with instant pudding. You get the picture. Around all this delicious food was the atmosphere for its consumption. Breakfast was always 6:20 to 6:27 a.m. Lunch was 12:10 to 12:25 p.m., and dinner was 4:43 to 4:58 p.m. Eating was always at the same time and for the same duration. Another layer to the dining experience was the emotional atmosphere surrounding this time, which was, to say the least, stressful. Every dinnertime for four or five years, I would knock something over or spill something. Maybe I made all the others stressed due to my clumsiness. Lunch involved the nuns policing the cafeteria aisles to be sure we were eating "right." If they deemed it not "right," we got hit. Great for digestion and relaxed eating.

Back then I never even thought about what I was eating, my diet, was it good for me or not, did I like the food or not. It was an unconscious act, even when I started to make my own food choices. And then I had a realization, a "aha" moment.

Small western Pennsylvania towns in the early 70s were pretty much homogeneous, at least the small streets of Carbon, Pennsylvania, where I lived were. Everyone was white and Catholic, attending the same school and church. By high school, I was transferred to the big township school, called Hempfield. Yes, prior to the cannabis ban, hemp was a major U.S. crop. There were hippies and Protestants there, and I made acquaintances of both. One such person, she even may have been Methodist or Jewish, told me that veal was actually baby calf. No, I thought, I didn't want to eat a baby calf. This led immediately to a brain cascade of other animals I didn't want to eat. Cows? No. Lamb? No. Pig? No. The questions and answers intuitively continued until, to summarize, I decided to eat no large mammals and no small mammals, like rabbits or possums. Then, how about birds? Turkeys, chickens, pheasants. The answer was again intuitively no. Then on to fish. How about crustaceans, shrimps, scallops, clams etc.? The answer was okay. This all happened in a flash. I was pretty much, for all intents and purposes, now called a vegetarian, or as my family and other folks would state, a weirdo.

From that inspirational moment, I never ate those animals again. There was no forethought, hind thought, or research; nothing. It was an internal knowing that poured forth from my consciousness from one statement, "Veal is baby calf."

That was about forty years ago, and my bewildered parents' predictions about my imminent bouts with scurvy and beriberi (vitamin deficiencies) have not come to pass. In fact, the more I read about the treatment of animals, slaughterhouse conditions, preparation and handling of meat and meat products, and the numerous health concerns related to constant meat eating, the more thankful I am that I listened to the inner wisdom that burst forth that day when I became "one of those."

Believe me, I'm not advocating that everyone should be a vegetarian. I'm passing this along because I know that it is extremely important for you to find your own inner wisdom when it comes to what your particular body needs and wants. Don't listen to anyone else. My blood type is "O" and according to Dr. Peter D'Adamo, author of *Eat Right for Your Type*, I should be on a high meat diet if I want to feel good and stay healthy. But who knows what is best for me, an author (even one I think is brilliant) or my inner wisdom? Now the other part of listening to your body's wisdom is making sure that what you are doing is working for you. How do you feel?

There's a huge list in our heads of what we should and shouldn't eat: big breakfast, dinner always, carbo load before activities, regular small meals, don't eat between meals, feed a cold and starve a fever, starve a cold and feed a fever. You get the drift. So, what if you threw out all of these notions and lists and ate what and when your body wanted. Yes, your unique body. What if your breakfast was just a protein drink, with some veggies mid-morning, a huge lunch, and no dinner? What if you were a vegetarian who didn't eat fruit because you didn't like fruit? Or what if your favorite staple was steak enjoyed after seven p.m.? Any of this is fine if (and this is the big if) it sustains you and makes you feel healthy and vibrant, with a good weight and energy level.

The bottom line is, the healthier you are, the more you are able to hear what your body needs. And at this point in your program, all you need to do is listen.

SUPPLEMENTS

It's blood-testing time! Now that you've been cleaning up your act and feeling better, it's time for a blood test to see if there is anything else you may need. You can do a screening panel to check for hidden bacteria, viruses, or yeast, along with iron levels. Plus, you can do an extended panel to evaluate particular nutrients, such as Vitamin D levels and kidney and liver enzymes. There are also hormonal tests you can get done, like estrogen and testosterone. Many of these will entail a twenty-four hour urine collection, which is exactly what it describes. You get a big red jug, and every time you pee, you pee into the jug. Just hope it doesn't start to overflow when you are mid-stream. That can get messy.

Where can you go to get these tests, or even to find out which ones are appropriate for you? If your primary care physician does not perform these test or if it isn't their field of expertise, do a little research for your area and find one that is familiar with ordering and interpreting your lab results.

Traditionally, medical doctors are trained to get a sick or dying person stabilized, which is very good thing. Unfortunately, what they are now dealing with are lifestyle diseases, such as heart disease, obesity, and diabetes. If these issues were caught and prevented earlier in life, many of them would not manifest into full-blown diseases. The patients need to see a wellness practitioner to stay well. So find someone who knows about alternative treatments or even see a nutrition/wellness practitioner. Chiropractors, acupuncturists, naturopaths, and nurse practitioners are all licensed healthcare providers who may be able to order these tests, and, even more important, interpret the results for you. Remember to maintain your daily vitamin supplements.

EXERCISE

It's time to check in on your exercise routine. How are you doing? Are you consistent? Are you getting bored? Or are you loving it so much that you now are exercising four to five times a week, mixing it up with some cardio and strength-training plus an everyday stretching routine? On the weekends, you're active, with fun stuff like biking, hiking, canoeing, water skiing, cross-country skiing, all of those things you just dreamed of doing. But now you are in much better shape because of your exercise routine, dietary changes, and supplements. And you are exercising longer and with more frequency.

You know, I've got four big dogs, and a bag of their food weighs twenty-eight pounds. This is a little heavy and cumbersome for me to lug out to the car and into the house once a week. Now can you imagine strapping on that twenty-eight pounds and carrying it around with you twenty-four hours a day, seven days a week, while feeding it, keeping it warm, and metabolizing it? Can you imagine how tired and sore you would be hiking with a backpack full of an extra twenty-eight pounds? No wonder the overweight and obese want to sit on the couch. I want to sit just thinking about it. And every pound you lose, you will feel lighter and lighter. Did you know that one extra pound of weight puts four extra pounds of pressure on the knees? That means that if you are ten pounds overweight every step you take puts forty extra pounds of pressure on your knees. (Arthritis Foundation). Things will become easier to do, and your stamina and energy level will increase. Life is going to look a little or a lot better. And you only have to thank yourself for it!

SUMMARY OF PHASE III

- **Diet:** Experiment with food elimination/rotation to ascertain which specific ingredients make you feel wonderful and which ones make you feel crummy. Then there is fine-tuning of your own innate knowing of which foods, diet, dining times, etc. work best for you.
- **Supplements:** Time to fine-tune what is optimal with specific blood panels and perhaps urine tests.

- **Exercise:** Being consistent, and changing up your exercise programs to keep them fresh and fun. Increasing the amount you exercise to four to five times/week and throwing in some extraneous activity, just for the fun of it.

TIME FRAME

You'll want to continue doing this routine of fine-tuning your diet and exercise routine for approximately three to four months. Additionally, you will continue your supplements and add any additional supplements, depending on the results of your blood and/or urine results.

What comes after this? Life, liberty, and more happiness. You have done the work. Now your great efforts and courage to change are here and now, and your rewards are your healthy and vibrant body and mind. Many people who have changed their lifestyles confess that they now feel better than they did twenty, thirty, or even forty years ago.

Ladies, isn't it great to see your new and improved version of your partner, who is now cleaning the garage, interested in new projects, and even may be planning your great new adventure together? Congratulations!

SOME MORE HELPFUL HINTS AND SUGGESTIONS TO ADD TO YOUR SUCCESS:

FOOD PLANS

Because it is difficult to initiate changes in dietary regimes, here are some simple guidelines along with weekly meal plans for PHASE I. By PHASES II and III, you will be fine-tuning and writing your own, depending on your unique body's requirements.

All food should be organic and definitely all meat and animal foods should be hormone and chemical free. No plastic containers, and, if your research supports it, no GMO!

BREAKFAST

Breakfast should contain protein that is easy to digest. Avoid processed carbohydrates for breakfast. If you're wondering what a processed carbohydrate food looks like, picture the all-American Continental breakfast and that's most of it: toast, cereal, waffles, pancakes, muffins, Danish. Skip all of that. I recommend a protein drink that is organic and soy-free. Protein will stay with you longer, so you don't dump your blood sugar two hours later and want another processed carbohydrate food. The overall proteins are fish, chicken, turkey, eggs, seafood, nuts, beans, legumes, and seeds. A good mid-morning snack could be peanut butter and celery, cheese and carrots, or hard-boiled eggs.

LUNCH

In other countries, people actually take hours for lunch, not fifteen minutes wolfing down some fast food. If you can, take time to eat, enjoy, and digest your lunch. Your car is going to be so much cleaner because you now aren't using it as your roving dining room. It's best, if you can't be at home, to have something prepared and take it with you to the office or your work. You know you are going to want to eat lunch, so plan ahead. I love lunch! When I was a child and spending time at my grandparents' house, they had their biggest meal at lunch. My grandfather worked from three to eleven, so lunch was the main meal, and my grandmother would pack up the leftovers in his "lunch pail." They would do this most days of the week after a light breakfast. I liked this schedule, and in my adult life, I have emulated this eating schedule. Getting off of work at six p.m. and still having to work out for at least an hour and then dog-feeding and chores would have me eating dinner about eight o'clock at night. Usually I will just have nothing or maybe a light snack before relaxing a little and going to bed. For me, the worst feeling is going to bed on a full stomach. I have nightmares. This works for me. You'll figure out what works best for you.

DINNER

Well, if you haven't earned it, you don't get to eat it! That's a basic rule. If you ate heartily throughout the day and did nothing much but sit at your desk, you don't get to gorge yourself at dinnertime. In fact, you get to go to bed with just a snack in your tummy. However, if you ate lightly throughout the day and did your exercise regime, you get to have dinner, but not too much.

WATER, DRINK IT

But don't drink water out of any plastic containers. Be sure that you drink plenty of water. Now I have heard so many times, "I don't drink water. I don't like the taste. I drink tea or coffee, but isn't that the same?" No, water is water and juice is juice; coffee is coffee; tea is tea, and sodas are sodas. Get the picture? If you don't like the taste of water put a little squeeze of fresh lemon in it or a fresh strawberry to add some flavor, but do drink it down. We've all heard the recommendation for drinking water: eight eight-ounce glasses a day, giving the average person sixty-four ounces of water daily. Who makes these recommendations? Seems to me that the amount of water your body requires is fairly unique. And it will fluctuate daily, even hourly, depending on so many factors, such as climate, activities, food consumption, age, health status. So many factors. When you're thirsty, drink, and even before you get thirsty, especially if you know you'll be sweating. Ah, your kidneys are going to love you!

Guys, I heard that you don't want to drink too much water because then you are up all-night peeing. This isn't so much due to the water consumption but enlargement of the prostate. People with bladder-control issues, like new mothers and elderly mothers, also don't like to drink water because they can't control their peeing. Drink the water, and get an adult diaper. If you don't get enough water, your system won't work correctly. We are ninety-eight percent water. We are mostly a sloshing bag of fluid and electrolytes. One sign that you are not getting enough water is fatigue and headache. So before you have another Tylenol with the next cup of coffee, try a couple of glasses of water and see what happens.

Here's a quick test to see if you need water. Pinch and pull up the skin on the back of your hand. It should fall back in place within five seconds. If not, go get some water. Notice I didn't mention the word dehydrated. Dehydration is a severe medical condition that needs immediate attention, and, of course, water. Don't you even let yourself get to that stage of needing fluids. Drink the water.

SNACKS CAN BE KILLERS

Let me tell you, snacks and random eating are about the worst problems in the food category. Snacks and extraneous food between meals, I think, are the biggest contributors to lifestyle health problems. Maybe that is because snack foods that are accessible, inexpensive, and "hit the spot…bing, bing, bing" are terrible for you: candy bars, salty fatty fried chips, cookies, etc. It's much easier to find a chocolate bar than an organic carrot. When I am grocery shopping, there's this phenomenon that occurs. If I don't put it in the cart, I don't buy it, and it won't somehow manage to make it into my pantry and into my mouth. Isn't that mysterious? Now, every once in a while, a sneaky bag of potato chips somehow jumps off the shelf into my cart, puts on an invisibility cloak (that somehow the cashier is immune to), and makes it home safe and sound with me. "Wow," as I go into the pantry later that night. "How in the world did those crafty potato chips get here again?" Unless you are like Goldilocks and are raiding your neighbor's fridge, if you don't buy it, it won't be in your house, and you won't eat it. So be very careful of what you put into your grocery cart. Oh, and be careful of those jumping chips and other migrating snack foods. It's amazing to go to other countries and look at their snacking patterns. They don't have them. Snacks are quite rare and unusual. If you miss a meal, you're pretty much out of luck until the next meal. Traveling abroad, I didn't see people walking around eating food or even driving around snacking in their cars, but I see that frequently in the States. It's like the car is the kitchen and the bathroom as well. I see a lot of personal grooming going on in the driver's seat.

SLEEP

Sleep, you need it to regenerate and rejuvenate your body and mind. It shouldn't be that difficult. My dogs do it all the time. Yet apparently it is a huge problem. Remember the anxiety issue of male menopause, when you're up in the wee hours of the morning worrying over something and anything? One of the reasons is that sleep patterns change with hormonal changes, and sleep is evasive. This causes the body stress and the cortisol hormone gets secreted and that causes the body to store fat. Stimulants are a big culprit so look at what you're taking during the day. Have a little bedtime routine, and stick with that routine. We did it as kids, and for our kids. And if it entails reading a brief bedtime story, then do it. If you get into bed and can't get the mind turned off, get up and do your routine again. This simple act will let the body know that it's time for bed. Deep breathing also is very helpful. Counting your breaths from ten down to one, and watching the breath go in and out of the lungs while counting them can change your physiology to a very relaxed state. Melatonin, a hormone the body secretes, can be added prior to bed. This will act as a sleep aid without the side effects of morning drowsiness.

I remember trying Melatonin initially when I was going through a stressful period of my life. Sometimes I'm not the smartest person when it comes to following my own clinical advice. I picked up a bottle at the health food shop and cracked it open. It was liquid, so, even without reading the label, I took a dropper, and then another and then another. I wanted to see what it would do to me. I barely made it home awake. I was so drowsy. Yep, I thought, this stuff really works. During that period of my life, I would put it on the nightstand next to my bed. I took some before bed, and if I woke up anytime in the night, I would take a dropper and go straight back to sleep. I never slept through my alarm and always felt refreshed when I got up. I love and appreciate that stuff and haven't used it in years, but when I needed it, it was very helpful. If you think Melatonin may be helpful for you, talk to your health consultant.

DIET

Just in case you are at a loss about what the heck would be a good weekly meal plan, initially, here is a sample. If you don't like it don't use it. It is a guideline, not a rule.

DAY 1

- Breakfast: Egg with mushrooms, celery with peanut butter
- Snack: Raw nuts and carrots
- Lunch: Chicken and salad (watch ingredients in that salad dressing)
- Snack: Boiled egg
- Dinner: Green salad and raw nuts
- Snack: Apple

DAY 2

- Breakfast: Tuna with cut veggies and raw nuts
- Snack: Peanut butter on celery

- Lunch: Cottage cheese and spinach salad
- Snack: Apple
- Dinner: Boiled egg and veggies
- Snack: Berries

Day 3

- Breakfast: Egg and apple
- Snack: Raw nuts
- Lunch: Tuna and cut veggies
- Snack: Raw nuts
- Dinner: Chicken salad and asparagus
- Snack: Hummus

DAY 4

- Breakfast: Egg with cheese chunks and raw almond and seeds
- Snack: Cheese
- Lunch: Salad and walnuts
- Snack: Carrots and celery
- Dinner: Soup and salad
- Snack: Raw nuts

DAY 5

- Breakfast: Peanut butter with celery
- Snack: Raw nuts
- Lunch: Fish and green salad
- Snack: Apple
- Dinner: Veggies and fruit salad
- Snack: Celery and hummus

DAY 6

- Breakfast: Fish and asparagus with butter
- Snack: String cheese
- Lunch: Collard greens and cheese
- Snack: Boiled egg
- Dinner: Kale salad with mixed greens
- Snack: Raw nuts and seeds

DAY 7

- Breakfast: Cottage cheese with berries and nuts
- Snack: Raw nuts
- Lunch: Hamburger patty with veggies
- Snack: Cheese and raw nuts
- Dinner: Fish and veggies
- Snack: Apple

After the first week, you can add a broader food menu, with yogurt, beans, more meats, avocado, and things like this. When you look at this sample menu, don't cry, or give up without at least trying it for a couple of days. At first, you may feel hungry and have cravings for your fast-food burgers, pizzas, potato chips, macaroni and cheese, and fettuccine Alfredo. That's okay. Feel the cravings, and eat this menu anyway. After the first week, you are going to feel so much better and you will want to stick with it. If you are getting a lot of back talk from your family, I understand. Hold your ground. You know they are going to go off and eat something yucky anyway. That's the nature of living where we live and in the time we live. You can get any type of food at any time of the day or night.

When my two stepsons were at my house, and I was cooking solo for the first time, I had no idea what to fix. I made mashed potatoes, veggies, and fish. I thought that safe enough. Well, about five minutes after the three of us sat down, the five-year-old picked up a huge spoonful of potatoes off his plate and winged them at me. Splat, dead hit on my face. Thinking I was going to kill him, I took several deep breaths as the two of them held their breaths to see what my reaction would be. Suddenly, I realized that to an outsider this scenario probably would look pretty funny, and I just started laughing at the situation. Oh, they both got no more dinner that night.

This was just a prelude to the next twenty years of food battles between the kids and me. I thought that they would be healthier if they cut back on their sugar intake. So, new rule: No sugar. One day I went into the garage and discovered, in a very crafty hiding place, a stack of empty candy bar wrappers. When the truth came out, they confessed that their grandmother felt so sorry for them, the poor deprived sugar-free mongrels, that she was supplying them with buckets of candy.

Even if most of my efforts to have them eat healthy failed, I know that I had to do what I did because that's what I believed would be best for them. And today, well, I'd like to report that my husband's and my hard work and diligence to their diet paid off and on their own they make stellar food choices, but I can't. They both eat the typical American diet and frequent fast-food joints. They both are presently overweight and could be in better physical condition. So do your best and don't be attached to the outcome when it concerns others, even those you love.

They will make their own decisions. All you can do is offer what you can and be the best example you can.

BLOOD WORK

Some of your family doctors, and even specialists, may not be familiar with the necessary tests to determine if a guy has low testosterone versus another medical condition, such as low thyroid or the onset of diabetes. Why is this? According to Abraham Morgentaler, M.D., physicians may not know exactly what tests to order. Or they will order the incorrect tests to diagnosis this condition. In medical school, promising doctors are taught to look for a potential brain problem or at the levels of testosterone in the blood. Yes, you would want to get a testosterone blood level count. But this is only part of the picture. There is the total testosterone level, which could then be broken down into free testosterone and testosterone that is tied up with other molecules and is not readily available. Think of them as your financial assets. You may look great on paper with home equity, 401(k), and retirement funds that you really couldn't liquidate into ready cash today. But you may be able to go to your bank and withdraw some money and have some available cash. That's how testosterone in the blood works. There is the total testosterone and then there is free testosterone, testosterone that is bound "lightly" to albumin, and testosterone that is "tightly" bound to a big protein (SHBG).

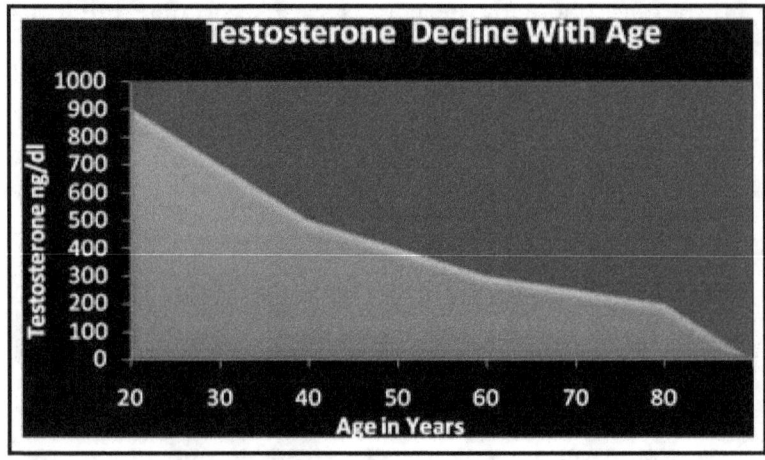

Source: New Agave Health Solutions for Men

If you only measured the total testosterone without measuring the free and lightly bound testosterone, then you aren't getting a good picture of what's really going on. You want to know how much of the "juice" is bio-available, or if you think of it in terms of money, how much is "liquid."

Remember that this is a syndrome. A syndrome is basically a collection of symptoms that fit together, like a puzzle, to form a diagnosis. You have to put all of the symptoms together: mental, physical, emotional, and sexual, plus the blood work evaluation. Then, from that information keep in mind the following: If it looks like a horse, smells like a horse, and sounds like a horse, it's probably not a zebra. It's probably a horse.

CONCLUSION

I hope you have enjoyed reading this book and that the suggestions and information presented can help you and your family to feel and function better and better with each passing year. If there are certain aspects to the program that don't jive with you and your family, simply pass on them. Do what you can. Do your best, and that will be good enough. My wish and hope for you and your family is health, love, and laughter.

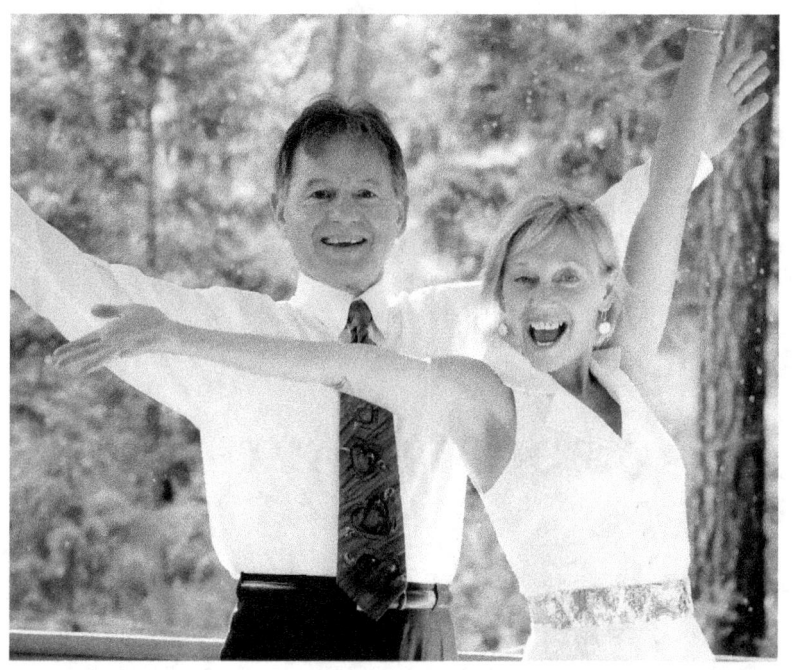

Thank you!

Dr. Patricia Skergan, D.C.

ABOUT THE AUTHOR

Dr. Patricia Skergan, D.C. holds a BS in Nutrition Science from Pennsylvania State University and a Doctorate in Chiropractic. She has been in private practice for twenty-seven years, most of those with her husband, also a chiropractor. Dr. Patricia is an A.C.E. certified group fitness instructor and personal trainer.

When not in the office or in the gym, she loves to send time walking her dogs, playing with her granddaughters, and enjoying outdoor activities.

End-Notes

---

[i] Sources: She-Economy, Ms. Smith Marketing, StartUpNation, ClickZ Inc. Girl Power Marketing, Catalyst, Forbes.

[ii] Pew Research Survey.

[iii] Dr. Todd Kashdan, *Huffington Post*; Thomas Joiner, "Lonely at the Top".

[iv] Travison *et al, Journal of Clinical Endocrinology and Metabolism*, 92, 196-204.

[v] *CDC National Vital Statistics Report*, Vol. 58, No. 8.

[vi] World Health Organization (WHO) Essential Medicines and Health Product Information Portal.

[vii] National Institute on Drug Abuse, May 2014.

[viii] The CDC used the NHANES (National Health and Nutrition Examination Survey) program: cdc.gov/exposurereport/pdf/fourthreport.pdf.

[ix] Gunther AL, Karaolis-Danckert N, Kroke A, et al, "Dietary protein intake throughout childhood is associated with the timing of puberty." *J Nutr* 2010, 140, 565-571.

Veldhuis JD, Roemmich JN, Richmond EJ, et al, "Endocrine control of body composition in infancy, childhood, and puberty", Endocr Rev 2005, 26, 114-146.

Wiley AS. "Milk intake and total dairy consumption: associations with early menarche in NHANES 1999-2004." PloS one 2011;6:e14685.

Annual Review of Nutrition 1991, 11, 325-53.

[x] *International Journal of Behavioral Nutrition and Physical Activity,* 2014, 11; *Harvard Health Publication*, May 22, 2013.